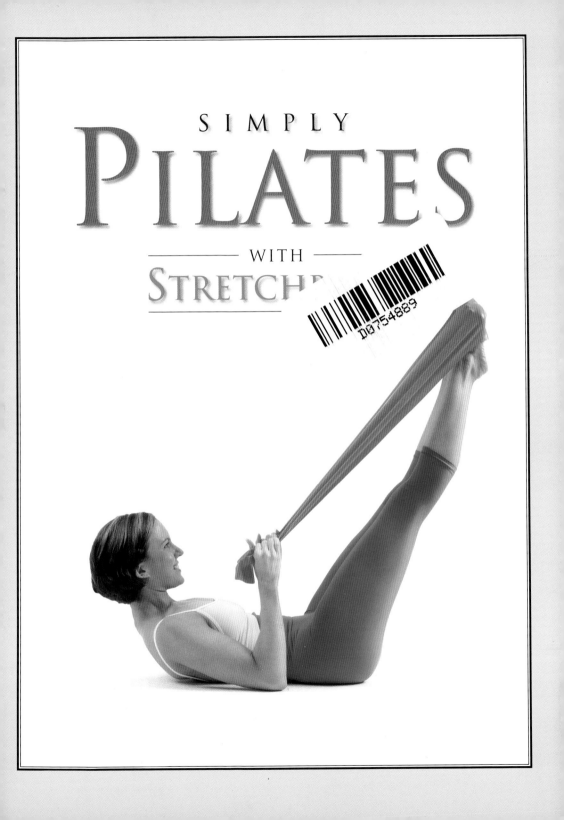

SIMPLY
PILATES

— WITH —
STRETCHES

Author: Jennifer Pohlman
Art Director: Karen Moores
Editor: Jane Keighley
Graphic Artist: Susie Allen
Photographer: Paul Broben
Assistant Co-ordinator: Rodney Searle

First published in 2005 by Hinkler Books Pty Ltd
45-55 Fairchild Street
Heatherton VIC 3202 Australia
www.hinklerbooks.com

Printed and bound in China
4 6 8 10 9 7 5
08 10 09 07

ISBN 1 7415 7533 8

CONTENTS

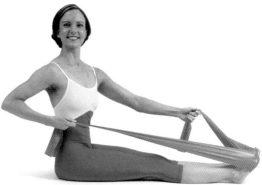

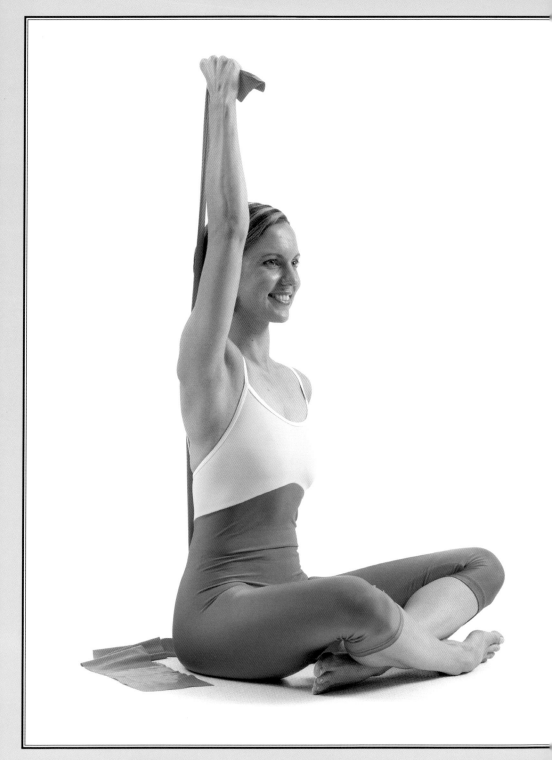

INTRODUCTION

In the early 1900s, German-born Joseph Pilates devised a system of movement which, when practised regularly focusing on quality of movement and alignment, will give you improved general fitness.

Pilates, in its true form, is a training regime based on the principles of refining physical motion. This exercise regime is gentle, effective and often subtle, requiring patience and consistency in order to achieve long-term benefits. The exercises were designed to be performed with exact technique and minimal repetitions, encompassing the less-is-more workout philosophy.

Joseph educated his students to be dedicated to the discipline on a daily basis, so mind and body were conditioned and the movement (much like martial arts or dance) was worked to perfection.

Joseph died in the 1960s but his exercise method evolved into various forms, with his original students dispersing to cities all over the world to establish their own training schools. Although the Pilates Method of body conditioning can vary greatly in 'what' it is and 'how' it is taught around the globe, the Pilates principles, which are the philosophy behind Joseph's exercises, are the common thread that binds the different Pilates schools. Physical therapists use the basis of Pilates postural concepts, along with modified versions of the movement sequences, for rehabilitating patients and the elderly.

At the other end of the spectrum, Pilates floor classes are becoming commonplace in gyms and fitness centres, varying by degrees of difficulty and dynamics. There are now an increasing number of Pilates exercise studios, predominantly in main cities, which host private and semi-private sessions so you can experience a full-body workout program using a combination of floor and equipment exercises.

Joseph originally developed the repertoire of floor exercises for the purpose of full-body conditioning, then later improvised with springs and pulleys to take the method to another level – inventing Pilates equipment. Integrating a stretchband into a Pilates floor workout can simulate resistance that is usually achieved on Pilates equipment.

His own exercise studio was situated in the same building as a major ballet company in New York City and he worked with the dancers to correct muscle imbalances, improve symmetry and eradicate poor movement patterns. He referred to his exercise system as The Art of Contrology and endeavoured to help people from all walks of life. Although he had devised choreographed movements for the purpose of full-body strengthening, he believed it was the principles with which his students executed the movements that were essential.

PILATES PRINCIPLES

Joseph's knowledge and experience of physical movement helped him devise a fusion of principles that epitomise a sensible approach to training the body for greater proficiency of movement. He believed an individual could train their body to perfect their daily movement patterns, whether they are an office worker or an athlete. If you embody these following powerful fundamentals, you will achieve the most from practising the Pilates technique:

- **Concentration** – visualisation and mental focus are essential to gain muscle control
- **Control** – quality movement is most beneficial and less harmful to joints and muscles
- **Centring** – the abdomen, lower back, hips and buttocks comprise the 'powerhouse' – the primary focus for strength, stability and 'core' control
- **Fluidity** – graceful, flowing motion is required, with no static, abrupt or rushed movements
- **Precision** – purposeful movement and good body alignment develops better muscle patterns for everyday activities
- **Breathing** – calm, rhythmic breathing assists muscle control and energises the whole system

Joseph was influenced by various physical disciplines, such as body building, boxing, diving, gymnastics and dance. Of course, these exacting sports require ultimate physical conditioning. They depend on strength, suppleness, control, precision, agility and the acquired understanding of movement quality and dynamics. Training the body for specific sporting manoeuvres requires consistent practise, allowing the individual to develop strength and efficiency in what

it is they need to do repetitively. Considering the extreme fitness usually required for such sports, it was apparent to Joseph how certain physical laws, or principles, needed to be followed in order to make the process possible. Fusing concepts of strength building with holistic life philosophies of Eastern origins, the principles aim to help people manage and improve their physical limitations. He developed a series of choreographed movements and personally instructed individuals through tailored training sessions ranging from gentle to rigorous exercise sequences. Not unlike an athlete training his body to execute movement

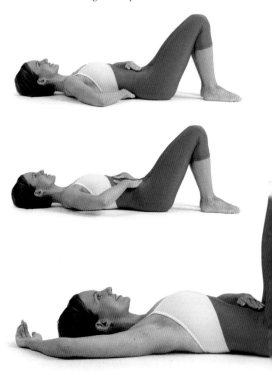

PILATES EQUIPMENT

with proficiency, the average person needs to ensure their body is fit for general living. Everyday movement – for example, carrying a washing basket full of wet clothes, climbing stairs repetitively, sustaining reasonable posture in front of a computer, maintaining spinal strength and stability while growing slowly while pregnant – all require a certain level of strength and endurance training. Everybody needs to develop and maintain optimal physical fitness for general living as well as any particular repetitive tasks they need to perform, to ensure their muscles and joints stay as resilient to wear and tear as possible. One-sided activities have an impact on our spines. Nursing a child on one hip, swinging a golf club and even driving a manual car creates muscular imbalance in our bodies. We need to condition our body to suit our needs. Pilates is a perfect body conditioning method for almost everybody to re-create muscle symmetry and strength.

It was essential to Joseph that the principles behind his Method were the central focus of each exercise, and when equipment was introduced it was an aid to challenge, modify or help facilitate movement which was otherwise not possible. He was adamant about the individual being in total control of their trunk and limbs. Appropriate muscle control needs to be used with, and against, the resistance of the springs. At no moment is the source of resistance to execute the movement for the individual. It is not about what a particular piece of equipment does for the body, but rather how an individual can achieve their optimum with the use of the equipment.

In a fully equipped Pilates studio, the equipment available to today's instructors is very close to that of Joseph's specially designed, spring-resistance based tables and carriages (on wheels, with pulleys and straps). A modern Pilates studio, which bases its teachings on Joseph's original work, can comprise of various exercise apparatus, as well as smaller pieces of equipment to challenge or assist the individual in their exercises. It is the above mentioned spring-loaded equipment that can be duplicated in effort and movement sequences on the mat with a stretchband.

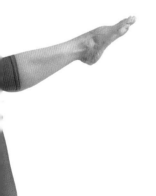

THE BENEFITS

Pilates principles are very adaptable to different mediums, which is why many medical and fitness professionals recognise the benefits of incorporating it into people's daily lives. Depending on an individual's fitness, co-ordination and musculoskeletal complications, anybody can perform Pilates exercises to some level and experience many different benefits. Due to the adaptability of Pilates, it is almost impossible to describe to someone who has not yet experienced its benefits, what it is.

Pilates is arguably of most benefit when taught individually to a person, or at most, up to four people at a time. The reason is that all bodies are unique – with different strengths and weaknesses – and Pilates exercises can be modified for you to achieve the most positive muscle patterning. This allows you to gradually build up to achieving a secure execution of pure Pilates sequencing. This process is fundamental when beginning Pilates, to prevent the development of bad habits in movement and to improve existing poor postural and movement habits.

Pilates is simply a sensible and correct method of physical realignment and strengthening – a fact well proven and documented through testimonials over the last 80–90 years. These include people devoted to practising Pilates for numerous reasons – general fitness, improved wellbeing, pain management, injury prevention, rehabilitation and post-natally, among others. From the athlete who uses Pilates to complement their other training, to the office worker who usually loathes exercise, regular Pilates sessions are a refreshing way to clear your mind and effectively strengthen and tone the body. The movement sequences are never boring and can increase in difficulty or intensity as you gain strength and perspective of the Method. Pilates can be many things and many ways of moving: it can become part of your lifestyle as it enhances your total wellbeing and improves your quality of living.

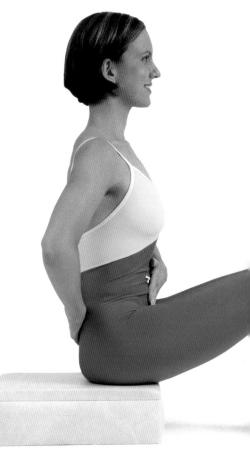

Practical Matters

Joseph was an advocate of the less-is-more philosophy when it came to exercise. In other words, the body is not forced or overworked to gain strength and endurance. In today's society of instant gratification, the masses are keen for any new fitness fad. Pilates, having the notable reputation for moulding sleek, strong physiques, is certainly no exception. However, there is a trade-off: commitment to routine practise and being very intuitive with your own body – taking it step-by-step and building on your physical successes with realistic progressions. Each exercise requires specific attention to detail – of both your alignment and your purpose of movement (i.e. what are you strengthening?).

Pilates is multi-functional as you introduce it to your fitness regime. Aiming for daily practise is ideal, even if it is only 15–20 minutes. Or realistically, schedule your practice sessions around your week's commitments and other sensible exercise. Pilates is a perfect addition to cross-training regimes.

Note: If you have a history of spinal, hip or shoulder problems, or if you are pregnant, seek advice from your medical practioner or visit a reputable Pilates studio prior to commencing these exercises.

Requirements

During your Pilates floor workout, the mat or carpet surface you lie on must be comfortable. However, if it is too soft, you will find it too difficult to maintain the natural curvature of your spine and your body will be forced to recruit other muscles to create a sense of stability. Your neck and shoulders must remain tension-free, so a small pillow or book may be required under your head. A low chair or a couple of phone books will create an appropriate height for you to sit on during the seated exercises if your hips and back lack the suppleness to sit completely upright. This is important when doing exercises that are specifically about correcting your posture. A cushion and bath-sized towel may be of assistance to you if your back or neck is compromised during any of the exercises. These options are explained in the content of the book.

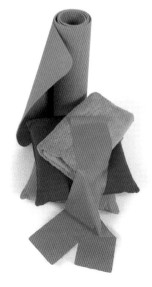

Centring & Breathing

The following three concepts are fundamental to developing good posture. Awareness of these concepts should be a prerequisite to any Pilates workout, and will ensure that you obtain maximum benefit from the exercises.

Breathing

Taking a moment to meditate on the rhythm of your breathing can be relaxing, release muscle tension, energise your whole system and ultimately draw your attention to your abdominal muscles. Take time to focus on how you breathe. Allow your ribs to soften and expand (side and back) as you breathe in, and merely relax as you exhale. In Pilates, we term this lateral breathing. The breathing exercise in this book will instruct you in co-ordinating breath and abdominal control. Over time this will feel fairly easy, allowing you to execute the Pilates exercises with greater ease and confidence.

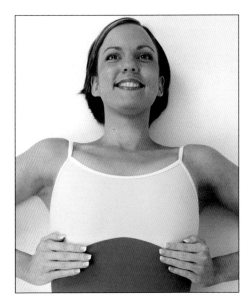

Neutral Pelvis

This is the most ideal position for you to strengthen your deep abdominal muscles in order to maintain or improve the stability of your spine. Lie on your back and relax your hip muscles. Usually the hip bones (iliac crests) and the pubic bone all form a parallel level with the floor. Maintaining a neutral position of the pelvis will automatically position the spine in its natural alignment. Before and throughout the exercises, the pelvis and spine must be stable in neutral, unless you are specifically rolling or mobilising your spine.

When your legs are in a tabletop (refer to page 25) position – as described in Hundred (refer to page 28), for instance – your pelvis should remain in neutral alignment with a *feeling* of anchoring your spine to the floor. The key is developing the abdominal and back strength to maintain this position. Don't forcefully push your lower back into the floor as this will cause you to overwork muscles unnecessarily.

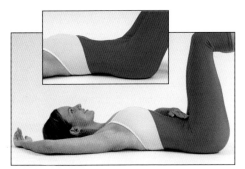

ABDOMINAL PATTERNING

Relaxed on your back is possibly the easiest position in which to establish awareness of correct abdominal activation. Place your hands on your lower abdomen and breathe normally. With your hips totally relaxed and maintaining your neutral pelvis and spine, merely sink or draw your abdomen away from your hands. The main thing to avoid is over-trying – never grip or clench your muscles. Subtleness is essential in creating an awareness of your deeper abdominal muscles. Your spine does not move, but try to visualise your belly and waist shrinking or being drawn in towards the front side of the spinal column itself. Because our deep postural muscles share nerve connections, lifting your pelvic floor muscles (while keeping your hips and buttocks relaxed) may assist in developing an intrinsic awareness of strengthening your core.

PREPARATORY NOTE
Pilates exercises – as well as associated modifications – require you to fuse the technical concepts of centring and breathing with general commonsense good posture. Know that the position of your head will affect your neck alignment. When you are lying on your back, your forehead and chin should be in a line parallel to the floor and your neck muscles should be free of tension. Place any pillow you may need under your head, not your neck. Remember, if you have pain or discomfort starting any of these exercises, discontinue and seek advice from a qualified professional.

During the execution of many Pilates exercises, you will be required to intensify this abdominal action, as well as squeeze your gluteal muscles (buttocks) a little. Take care not to bunch, or clench your abdominals in this case. Always aim for a flattening, scooping sensation with the abdomen while maintaining your neutral position.

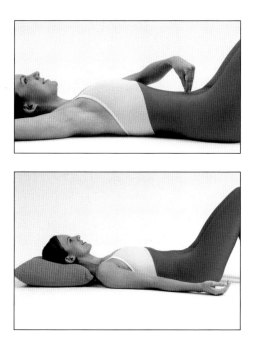

CENTRING & BREATHING *(continued)*

BREATHING EXERCISE

1 Lie on your back with your knees bent at a 90 degree angle, feet opposite your sitting bones (refer to page 63) and arms comfortably by your sides. This will be referred to as the preparatory position, because when you lie on your back, it is the simplest way of drawing your attention to full-body alignment.

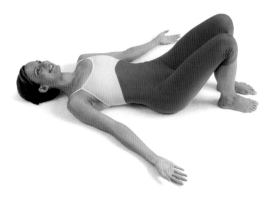

2 Assume a normal breathing pattern and be aware of maintaining your neutral pelvis position.

3 Keeping your neck and shoulders tension free and your hips totally relaxed, focus on your abdominal muscles gently bracing, or scooping. While you breathe, maintain the deep lower abdominal action without any spinal movement.

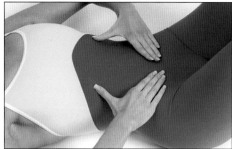

4 This concept can be practised while sitting. Wrap the stretchband around your ribcage so that you can have an immediate sensation of your ribs expanding and relaxing while you breathe. This may actually be very useful in creating awareness of your abdominal muscles engaging while you breathe freely.

NOTE

Visualisation techniques are often useful during Pilates exercises. Try imagining that your abdominal muscles are like a deep internal zip beginning near your pubic bone and going up the front of your spine towards your ribcage. Scoop, lift, zip, navel to spine, shrink, press down, draw in, inward and upward are all Pilates talk to help you visualise the action of your abdominal muscles for strengthening and stabilising purposes.

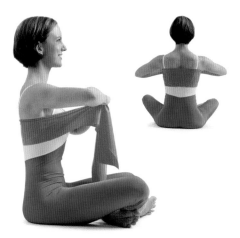

Scapula Movement

1 Lie on your back with the stretchband under your shoulder blades. Wrap it around the sides of your ribcage so you can hold the ends and reach your arms to the ceiling. While in the preparatory position, remember to focus on your breathing and abdominal technique. Relax your neck and shoulders.

2 As you inhale, push the stretchband towards the ceiling allowing your shoulder blades to move with your arms. Try to keep your ribcage, neck and head still and fairly relaxed.

3 Exhale using the muscles of your armpits and upper back to draw your shoulder blades back to their correct, flat alignment. Only move your shoulder blades enough to feel that you are creating a V formation with your back muscles. Keep your ribcage, neck and head still.

4 Repeat 5–6 times.

NOTE
Don't squeeze your shoulder blades together. Simply replace them to where you would consider them to be your best posture.

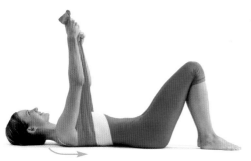

POSTURE AWARENESS

Purpose: *To mobilise and stretch your shoulders without straining your neck or moving your spine. These basic movements are preparatory exercises while you focus on the concepts of Centring & Breathing.*

ARM OPENINGS

1 Keep the stretchband under your upper back. Stay in the preparatory position and begin with your arms up towards the ceiling. Remember to breathe calmly and continue training your lower abdominals to gently shrink down towards the floor.

2 As you inhale, open your arms to the sides while you maintain correct alignment of the torso.

3 Exhale as you close your arms again. Relax your neck and keep your focus on your abdominal action and your shoulder blades being flat and stable.

4 Repeat 5–10 times.

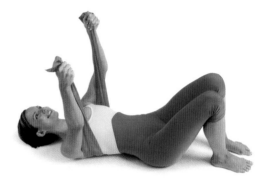

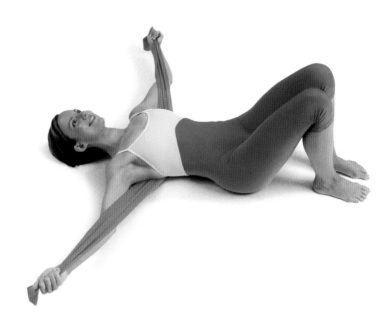

LAT STRETCH

1 Lie in the preparatory position and reach your arms towards the ceiling, holding the stretchband as though it was a pole. Breathe evenly and shrink through your stomach.

2 As you exhale, float your arms back to the floor behind you. Don't allow your ribs to arch off the floor. Maintain strong abdominal muscles as you lengthen your arms away from your ribcage.

3 Inhale as your arms return. Keep your shoulder blades flat and stable and relax your neck.

4 Repeat 5–6 times.

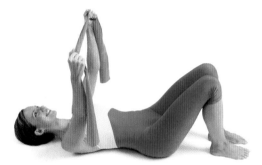

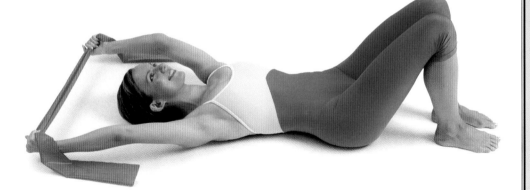

Posture Awareness *(continued)*

Pec Release

1 Stay in the preparatory position and keep the stretchband in your hands as though it was a pole. Bend your arms and rest them on the floor, placing the band above your head – taut but not stretched. Maintain your focus on ribcage and shoulder alignment so you don't compromise your neck, back or shoulder joints.

2 As you inhale, slide your arms along the floor further away from your head. Keep the distance between your hands about the same as the width of your elbows. There is no need to achieve straight arms because the purpose is to mobilise your shoulder joints while you maintain torso stability, and to keep your neck free of tension.

3 Exhale, bending your arms as they slide back towards you. You will possibly feel a stretch at the front of your shoulders and into your chest. Regardless, focus on the muscles of your upper back and stomach while you relax your neck and chest. Find a balance between not allowing your ribs to arch from the floor and maintaining a correct abdominal bracing action.

4 Repeat 5–6 times. Remember that the movement does not have to be big.

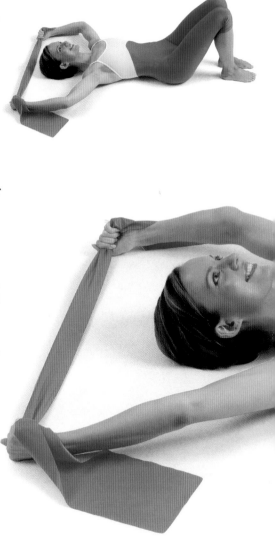

If this position is not achievable for your shoulders, upper back and neck, place your hands on your shoulders and let your arms relax out to the sides. Or stretch your arms out to the sides in a long position as far as comfortable to allow some stretch to occur across your chest and shoulders. Your neck should not experience any discomfort, your head should not be tilting backwards or your shoulders shrugging up towards your ears. If you are comfortable allow the stretch to continue for up to 1 minute.

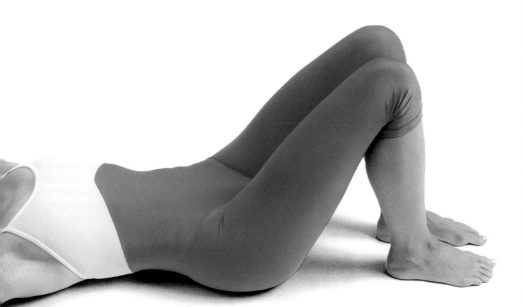

WARM UP

Purpose: *To integrate the concepts of better posture into exercises that begin to challenge your co-ordination as well as gently mobilise your spine. This will prepare your body for subsequent exercises.*

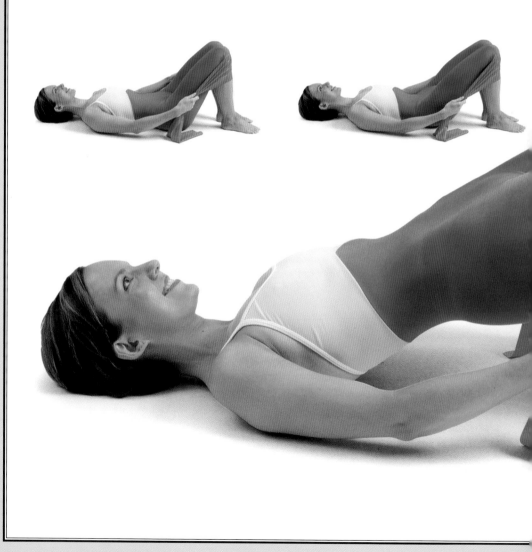

PELVIC CURL

1 Lie in the preparatory position with the stretchband around your shins, holding onto the ends with some resistance. Engage your deep abdominals. Inhale.

2 As you exhale, scoop your abdominals towards your lower back and curl your tailbone towards the ceiling. Peel your spine from the floor as if you are moving one vertebrae at a time. The stretchband may be slightly taut, reminding you of your shoulder posture. Relax your neck.

3 While at the peak of the lifted position, ensure it is your seat muscles (lower gluteals and hamstrings) lifting you and not your lower back. Breathe in laterally through your ribcage. Maintain tight abdominals and relax your neck.

4 As you exhale, reverse the roll gently as if you're imprinting the image of your spine, ribs and pelvis on the floor. Relax your hips completely at the end but maintain zipped abdominals.

5 Repeat 4–6 times.

WARM UP *(continued)*

CHEST LIFT

1 Start in the preparatory position and rest your head in the stretchband so that you can relax your neck muscles. Keep your focus on your shoulder blade stability, breathing and abdominal pattern. Don't allow your elbows to be too wide and keep your chin gently tilting down. Inhale.

2 As you exhale, roll your head and shoulders forward, flattening your abdominal muscles without moving your hips. Ensure the movement occurs through your ribcage and not through your neck or lower back.

3 Breathe in while you maintain a strong, broad abdominal bracing action.

4 Breathe out as you roll back to the floor. Take care not to release or clench your abdominal muscles.

5 Repeat 5–10 times.

6 Repeat remaining in the curled position while you continue to breathe. Take 5–10 full calm breaths while you focus on strong abdominals, relaxed thighs, stable shoulders and easy head and neck posture.

NOTE

The height of your curl forward is dependent upon the suppleness of your upper back and your abdominal strength. To achieve an easier position in which to develop abdominal strength without neck strain, place a cushion or rolled towel under your shoulder blades to assist your movement.

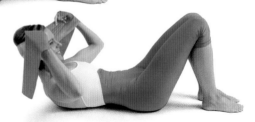

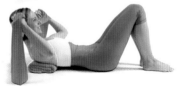

ROLL UP PREP

1 Sit with your legs bent in front of you. Keeping your feet flexed and about a tennis ball width apart, place the stretchband around the tops of your feet (toe and ball) and hold the stretchband with some resistance. Sit with fairly tall posture, but not rigid. Inhale.

2 As you exhale, gently roll your pelvis under so that your lower back becomes rounded. Roll away from your legs ensuring that your deep abdominal muscles pull in towards your spine.

3 Stop. Inhale. Maintain a deep scoop-up action with your lower abdominal muscles.

4 Remain still as you exhale – further deepening your abdominal scoop. Be careful not to collapse into your spine. Try to relax your neck and arms. Rather than overworking your shoulders, allow the stretchband to take some of your weight.

5 Inhale as you roll forward.

6 Repeat 4–6 times.

WARM UP *(continued)*

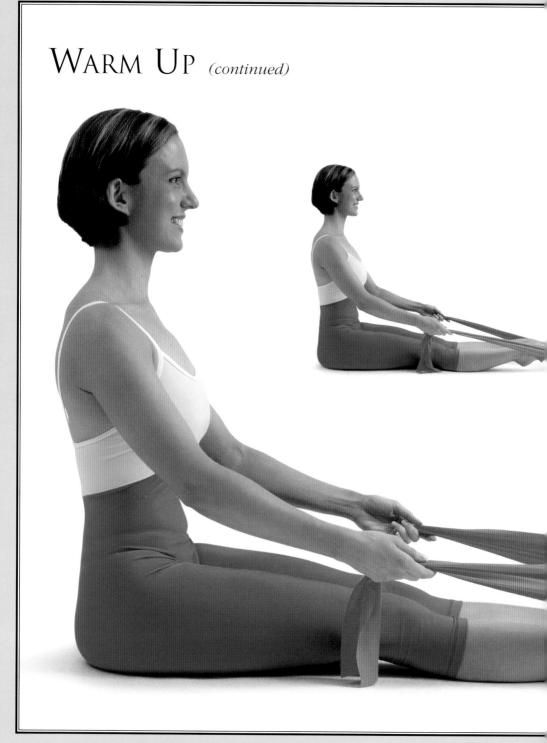

Footwork

1 Sit tall with your legs stretched out in front of you, slightly apart, and the stretchband around your toes and balls of your feet. Hold the ends of the stretchband with some resistance. Breathe normally.

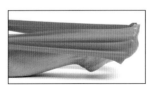

2 Stretch your legs completely and point your feet by way of moving your ankles first and then elongating the ends of your feet, through to the toes (metatarsals). Keep lengthening up through your lower back and stomach. Relax your neck and shoulders.

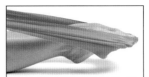

3 Flex your feet back up towards the ceiling beginning with your toes first, then your whole foot.

4 Repeat 10–20 times, depending on the strength and mobility of your feet, ankles and calves.

5 Maintain a lengthened ankle position and repeat just the metatarsal (toes and balls of your feet) movement for strengthening the underneath surface of your forefoot. Repeat 10–20 times.

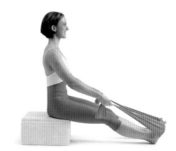

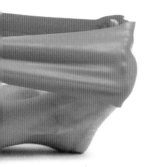

Note

This is the first exercise in your workout where you are sitting tall for a sustained period of time. Ensure you are sitting on your sitting bones, scooping up your abdominal muscles, and keeping your chest open so you can feel your postural muscles strengthen. Remember to sit on something higher if you are struggling to sit completely upright whilst on the floor.

PELVIC & SPINAL STABILITY

Purpose: *To realise how your core abdominal, hip and back muscles must work in order to keep your spine and pelvis in a natural alignment while your limbs move independently of your torso. This is essential to understand before embarking on traditional Pilates mat work.*

BEND & STRETCH

1 Lie in the preparatory position with the stretchband around the ball of one foot. Hold the ends with some resistance and place your elbows on the floor beside you. Ensure you maintain a neutral pelvis, stable ribcage and shoulder blades and shrink through your abdominals.

2 Exhale as you extend your knee, reaching your leg away from your torso. Maintain correct torso alignment and try not to involve your other leg.

3 Inhale as you bend your knee and return your leg to a tabletop position.

4 Repeat 5–10 times.

5 Keep the same foot in the stretchband and raise your other leg to tabletop, keeping your spine and pelvis stable and correctly flattening your abdominal muscles. Repeat the same exercise as you did with one leg extending in the stretchband. Your abdominal and hip muscles are challenged more since you have no feet on the floor. Keep your tabletop leg still, abdominals scooping, shoulders and ribcage stable, and breathe calmly.

6 Repeat 5–10 times.

7 Keep both legs in the tabletop position then extend one leg away from you, maintaining torso stability. Now, as one leg stretches, the other will bend and vice versa. Continue switching your legs while you focus on correct abdominals, breathing and leg alignment. Keep your knees a couple of inches apart and use your thigh and hip muscles.

8 Repeat 5–10 times.

9 Repeat all 3 variations with the stretchband around your other foot.

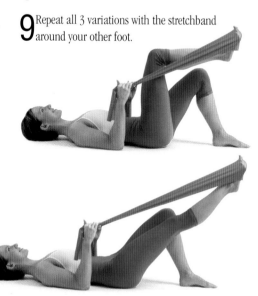

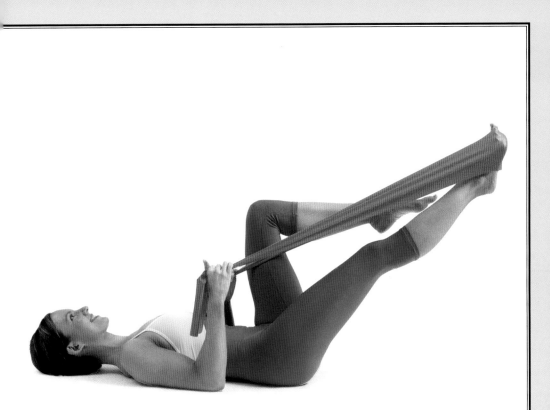

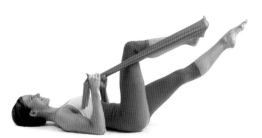

NOTE

The term tabletop refers to when one or both legs are in the air and bent at a 90 degree angle at both the hip and knee joints. The exact angle of this position will possibly vary between individuals according to your ability to stabilise your back with a secure abdominal pattern. The weight of your legs should be distributed down into your hip joints, or over your hip bones. You should feel no strain, but still keep the abdominal challenge reasonable.

If you struggle with the tabletop position, or cannot stop from clenching or bulging up your abdominal muscles, keep your feet on the floor or rest your feet on a chair until you are strong enough.

Pelvic &
Spinal Stability *(continued)*

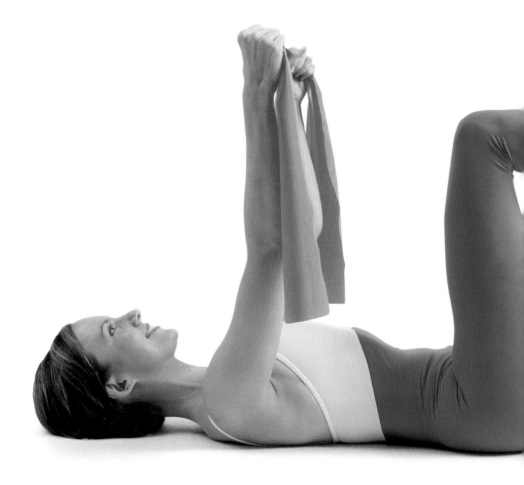

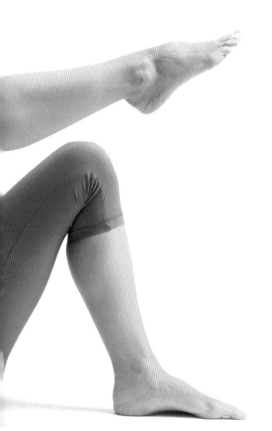

DEAD BUG

1 Begin in the preparatory position and hold the stretchband in both hands as though it was a pole. There is no need to create much resistance with the stretchband as this is just a guide for you to feel how symmetrical your neck, shoulder and ribcage areas are. Reach your arms to the ceiling and flatten your shoulder blades against the floor, relaxing your neck. Scoop and shrink your stomach towards the floor while maintaining a neutral pelvis. Lift one leg to tabletop.

2 As you breathe out, extend your leg from tabletop away from you and lower your arms towards the floor behind you. Only reach your limbs as far as you can so as to maintain correct torso alignment and stability.

3 Inhale, returning to the starting position.

4 Repeat 5–10 times, then swap legs and repeat.

PILATES FUNDAMENTALS

Purpose: *These exercises were traditionally the first exercises executed in a basic Pilates mat work sequence in order to prepare your body for subsequent abdominal work. Using a stretchband helps you achieve a better abdominal pattern and ensure smooth movement.*

HUNDRED

1 Lie on your back with your legs together in the tabletop position. Place the stretchband across your knees or shins and hold the ends in your hands by the sides of your hips.

2 Exhale as you curl your head and shoulders forward, similar to a Chest Lift position. Maintain correct abdominals, neutral pelvis and breathe calmly and smoothly as you begin pulsing your arms with small, quick movements.

3 Continue focusing on shrinking your waist and deep abdominal muscles, anchoring your pelvis still and flattening your shoulder blades while you aim for 10 full breaths.

4 Hold your arms still on your last breath in. Keep your centre strong and still.

5 Exhale as you rest.

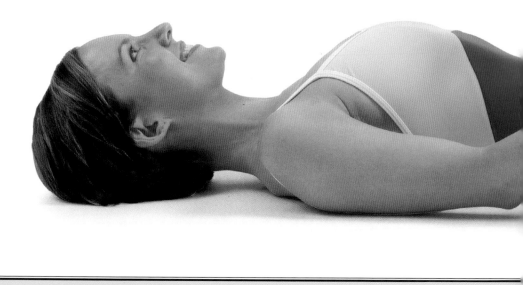

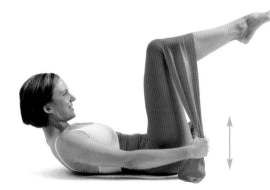

NOTE

Ultimately, the Hundred exercise should entail the co-ordination of 5 arm pulses each inhale and 5 pulses each exhale. This is to encourage optimal lung capacity while challenging the endurance of your abdominal muscles. So that you don't hyperventilate, start with less pulses per breath and build on that as you gain control and co-ordination.

Pilates Fundamentals *(continued)*

Roll Up

1 Sit with your legs bent in front of you, slightly apart, and the stretchband around the balls of your feet. Hold the stretchband relatively loosely, sit tall through your waist and lift your abdominals. Inhale.

2 As you exhale pull your lower abdominal muscles in towards your spine so that you roll easily backwards. Gradually roll to the floor as though you are gently kneading each section of your spine into the mat. You must feel anchored to the floor by your buttocks so you can move fluidly through your spine.

3 While you lie on the floor breathe in, focusing on the stability and symmetry of your torso. Keep your deep abdominal muscles engaged inward and upward towards your lower back.

4 As you exhale, nod your chin gently and roll towards your legs as though you are peeling yourself off the floor. Remember to anchor your hips to the floor and emphasise your abdominals into your lower back to ensure that you roll properly, using your legs as little as possible.

5 Repeat 3–4 times, then again with straight legs.

Note
While you are learning to articulate your spine and roll properly through your lower back with abdominal control, bent knees are likely to be more suitable to ensure the safety of your spine. Remember also that the stretchband is like training wheels for you to successfully roll up and down with a sense of length, strength and control throughout your spine and abdominal muscles.

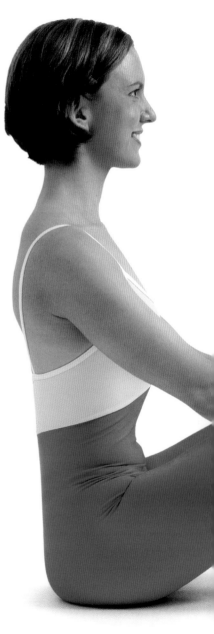

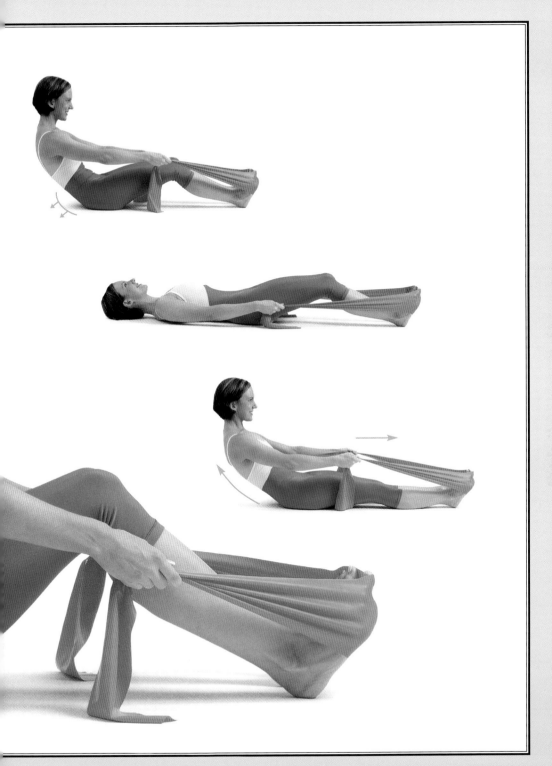

Pilates Fundamentals *(continued)*

Leg Circles

1 Lie on your back with the stretchband around one foot and the other leg either bent or straight on the floor. Hold the ends of the stretchband with some resistance and place your elbows on the floor beside you. Maintain a neutral and well-anchored spine and pelvis. Lengthen your (stretchband) leg towards the ceiling, maintaining correct torso placement. Don't allow your knees to turn in or out – they must line up with your ears or shoulders.

2 Draw a circle in the air with your foot. Your whole leg should move as this is an exercise to mobilise your hip joint while you keep your pelvis still and abdominals strong. Start your circles across your body first (towards your other hip) and exhale each time your leg raises back towards your body.

3 Repeat 6–10 times, then reverse the direction. Repeat both directions with your other leg.

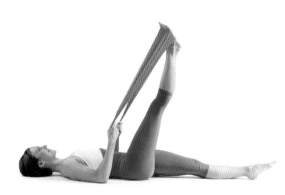

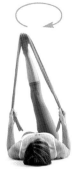

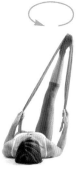

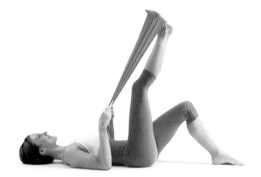

NOTE

Feel your hip, abdominal and upper back muscles bracing to keep your body still and strong while you execute your circles. Lengthen your other leg along the floor to assist you in being stable. Remember to only make the circles as big as you can and keep your torso still. Bend your raised leg if you are struggling to maintain a neutral pelvis.

PILATES FUNDAMENTALS *(continued)*

ROLLING PREP

1 Sit with your legs bent and very close to your body. Your feet should be together, but not necessarily your knees. Hold the stretchband out in front of your legs as though it was a pole. Don't stretch it greatly. Focus, instead, on a rounded body while drawing your shoulder blades flat and keeping your abdominals scooped strongly.

2 As you exhale, pull your deep abdominal muscles in towards your lower back, causing your hip bones to roll very slightly away from your thighs.

3 As you inhale, relax.

4 Repeat 5–6 times.

5 Repeat again with the stretchband across the front of your thighs. As you draw your stomach away from your thighs, pull the stretchband towards your feet to create an opposing resistance.

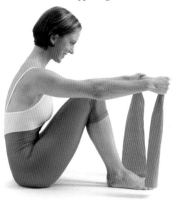

NOTE

In this exercise it is essential to move with subtlety
and focus on releasing your thigh muscles as you
engage your very deep lower abdominal muscles.
There should barely be any movement as this is
merely a preparatory exercise for rolling your spine
on the floor and maintaining a round back. You
are actually refining how you use your abdominal
muscles to flex your spine into a round shape.
If you find your hip muscles are cramping and
you're struggling with your lower back, sit up
on a couple of books.

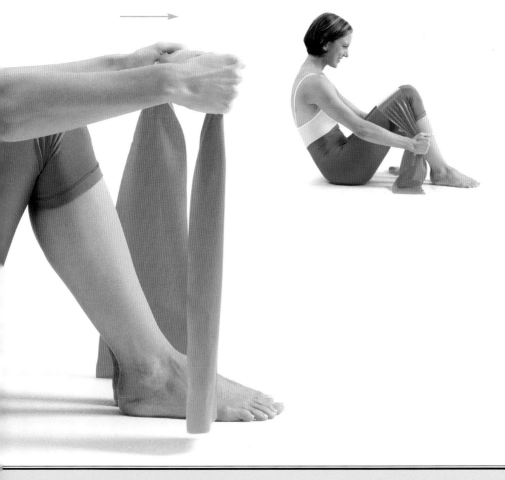

INTERMEDIATE ABDOMINALS

Purpose: _To further challenge your abdominal strength and endurance as you become secure with the Pilates warm up and fundamental exercises. While aiming for fluid, co-ordinated movements, you must always emphasise the placement, symmetry and stability of your pelvis, spine, ribcage and shoulder blades._

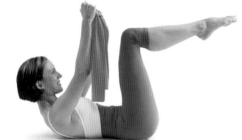

SINGLE LEG STRETCH

1 Lie on your back with your legs at tabletop and your head and shoulders curled forward. Hold the stretchband like a pole, reach your arms to the ceiling above your waist and flatten your shoulder blades and abdominals. A neutral and anchored pelvis is essential.

2 Breathe out as you extend one leg away from you and inhale as it returns.

3 Repeat 10–20 times, alternating legs.

NOTE
Breathe broadly, ensuring you are flexing forward from the base of your ribcage, flattening your shoulder blades and pressing your lower abdominal muscles deep towards the floor. Do not move your body during the leg extensions.

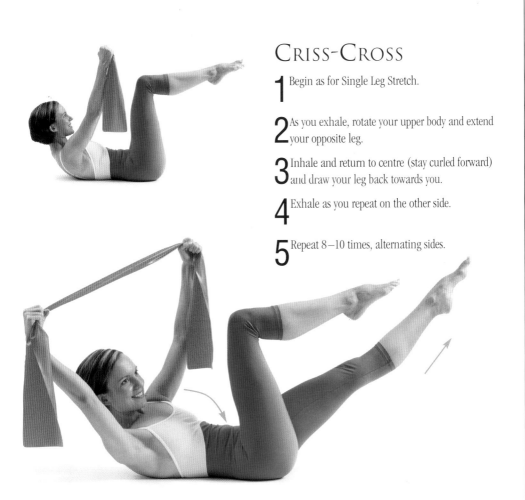

CRISS-CROSS

1 Begin as for Single Leg Stretch.

2 As you exhale, rotate your upper body and extend your opposite leg.

3 Inhale and return to centre (stay curled forward) and draw your leg back towards you.

4 Exhale as you repeat on the other side.

5 Repeat 8–10 times, alternating sides.

NOTE

Ensure you only rotate your ribcage as far as you don't lose the flexed forward strength. Your pelvis should remain neutral and anchored still throughout, and your abdominal muscles should be pressing towards your spine constantly.

INTERMEDIATE ABDOMINALS *(continued)*

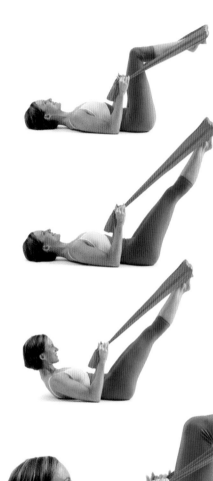

DOUBLE LEG STRETCH

1 Lie on your back with the stretchband around both feet. Don't allow your legs to relax. Keep your feet slightly apart so that you engage your hip muscles. Hold the ends of the stretchband and place your elbows at your sides. Start with a neutral spine and pelvis and your legs at tabletop.

2 Brace through your deep abdominals and, as you exhale, stretch your legs up and away from your torso. Only go as far as you can, maintaining correct alignment and abdominal work.

3 Inhale as your legs return. Maintain flat abdominals and stable ribs and shoulder blades.

4 Repeat 5–6 times.

5 Repeat all, curling your head and shoulders forward as you extend your legs, and bending your legs as you lie down.

6 Repeat all, maintaining a curled Chest Lift position – moving your legs only.

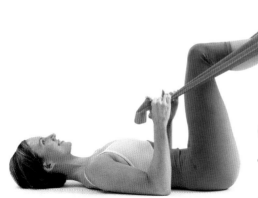

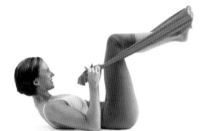

CO-ORDINATION

1 Start as you did for Double Leg Stretch.

2 As you exhale, curl your head and shoulders forward maintaining your legs at tabletop. Keep a strong centre, neutral pelvis and flat shoulder blades.

3 Inhale as you stretch your legs up in front of you.

4 Exhale, separate your legs into the stretchband and draw them together again.

5 Inhale. Bend your knees and lie down with control.

6 Repeat 5–10 times.

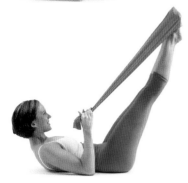

NOTE

Apart from co-ordinating controlled movement and breathing, it is essential that you do not move your spine and pelvis when you separate your feet and legs. This is a challenge of your pelvic stability when your legs go in separate directions.

Scapula Stability & Back Extension

Purpose: *To strengthen your shoulder and middle upper back muscles for better posture. These exercises must not cause strain to your lower back and neck.*

Back Extension With Arms

1 Lie face down with your arms bent at a 90 degree angle next to your shoulders. Hold the stretchband loosely in your hands. Your pubic bone and lowest ribs should be anchored to the floor – make them your anchor points. Gently draw your shoulders back and hover your head and shoulders away from the floor, just enough to feel your middle upper back muscles engage. Zip your abdominals from pubic bone to navel, shrinking your stomach up to your spine, without moving your spine.

2 As you balance on your anchor points, exhale stretching the stretchband and lightly grazing your little fingers along the floor. Keeping your stomach up and your shoulders back is important. Try to relax your neck.

3 Inhale as you allow the stretchband to retract, ensuring that you maintain upper back and abdominal strength. Don't go round shouldered and don't be tempted to lift your back too high.

4 Repeat 3–4 times before relaxing to the floor. Execute 3 sets in total.

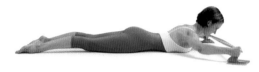

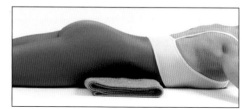

Note

This exercise focuses on the muscles of your upper back and shoulders to prepare you for more advanced Pilates back strengthening. Try to resist shrugging, rounding or squeezing your shoulder blades together. If you feel your lower back overworking, you are possibly lifting too high or not lifting your abdominal muscles. You may need to place a folded towel under your abdomen to help support your spine.

BREASTSTROKE

1 Start as you did for Back Extension With Arms. The same principles apply throughout this exercise. The difference is that you start with your arms further forward on the floor. Maintain your abdominals and draw your shoulders back to feel your middle upper back engage. Anchor your ribs to the floor as you lift your chest slightly. Breathe in.

2 As you exhale, stretch the stretchband so that your arms reach wide and arch your upper back further from the floor. Remember that you are bending from your upper back, not lower. Keep your arms slightly rotated so that the palms of your hands almost face each other.

3 Inhale. Allow the stretchband to retract and slowly return your chest to the floor with your arms moving forward again.

4 Repeat 5–6 times. Also try reverse breathing to challenge your muscle control.

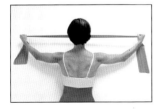

NOTE
Don't crane your neck to look up – imagine lengthening the area from the back of your ears to the top of your head. Keep your knuckles hovering lightly along the floor, keeping a sensation of opening your chest, while you shrink your abdominals up.

SIDE STABILITY & HIP STRENGTH

Purpose: *To challenge your balance and strengthen your stomach, back and hip muscles. Developing the ability to move your leg without moving your pelvis and spine requires co-ordination and causes your stabiliser muscles to work hard.*

LEG PRESS

1 Lie on your side with your underneath leg slightly bent for better balance. Place the foot of your top leg inside the stretchband and hold the ends of the stretchband in one hand, next to your hip. Brace your abdominals as though they were a corset holding you together. Take care not to rotate your spine.

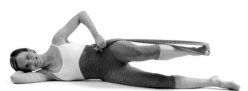

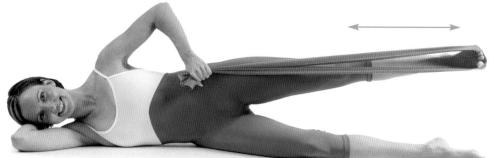

2 As you exhale, push your foot into the stretchband and lengthen your leg away, in line with your body. You may aim your foot slightly behind your body in an effort to feel your gluteal muscles (the back of your hip) more. Do not arch your back.

3 Inhale, allow the stretchband to loosen and your knee to bend. Keep your knee at hip height so you don't go knock-kneed.

4 Repeat 6–10 times each side.

NOTE
Balance on the underneath hip rather than your thigh and keep lengthening your top hip down towards your foot (even as your knee bends). Visualise the movement as being similar to propelling yourself off the side wall of a pool and through the water, using your hip and thigh muscles to achieve a straight and streamlined body. Scoop your abdominals constantly.

SMALL CIRCLES

1 Stay on your side as you were for Leg Press. Keep your top leg stretched straight with your foot in the stretchband. Emphasise the lengthening of your top hip towards your heel constantly and balance on your underneath hip rather than your thigh and scoop your abdominal muscles.

2 Breathe calmly as you execute fast, small circles with your top leg. Maintain your leg at hip height and try not to let the circles go too far forward or backwards. They must be compact and your pelvis and spine must stay as still and strong as possible.

3 Repeat approximately 10 circles in each direction, on each side.

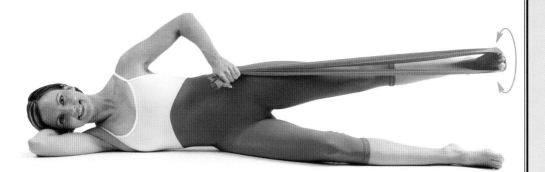

SHOULDER & ARMWORK

Purpose: *To strengthen your shoulder, arm, chest and upper back muscles for general strength and better posture.*

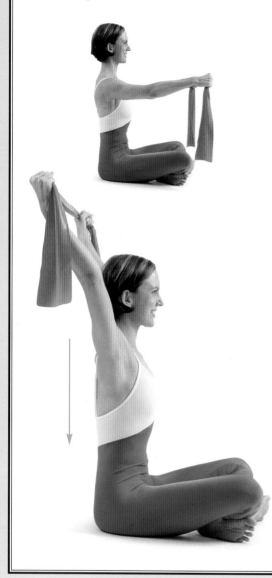

NOTE

If you suffer from acute neck problems, some of this armwork may overuse muscles that are already tight and associated with your pain. Seek professional advice regarding appropriate neck stretches and postural strengthening exercises suitable for you.

SHOULDER STRETCH

1 Sit up, cross-legged, and hold the stretchband as though it was a pole. Lengthen your waist and ensure you are sitting on your sitting bones. Relax your neck and shoulders, pull your stomach to your spine and breathe normally.

2 Keep your arms relatively straight and raise them to the ceiling. Your primary focus should be on good posture and allowing your shoulders to drop away from your ears. Be careful not to arch your back in order to raise your arms higher.

3 Once your arms are up, allow them to move slightly further behind you to stretch your shoulder muscles. Breathe normally and hold momentarily before returning your arms down in front of you.

4 Repeat 2–3 times.

NOTE

For all sitting exercises over the next few chapters, your lower back must be comfortable. Please sit on a couple of phone books or a chair if it helps you to sit straighter.

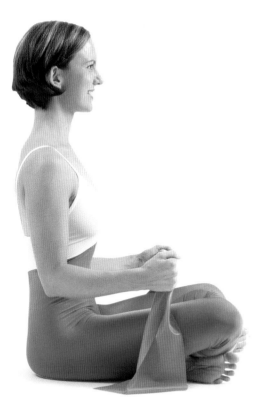

ROTATOR CUFF

1 Sit tall, holding the stretchband with your hands about shoulder width apart. Lengthen up through your waist and pull your shoulders back, without arching your back.

2 Exhale, rotating both shoulder joints as though they were hinges opening at the front. Don't necessarily squeeze your elbows against your body, but keep your upper arms completely vertical throughout the exercise. Keep a sense of your chest being open.

3 Inhale. Relax but keep a good shoulder position.

4 Repeat 10–12 times at a steady pace.

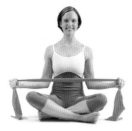

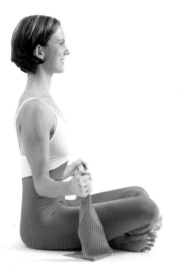

NOTE
Keep a strong wrist position, thumbs on top of the stretchband with the back of your hands facing outward. You should feel the muscles at the back of your shoulder more than those at the front.

SHOULDER & ARMWORK *(continued)*

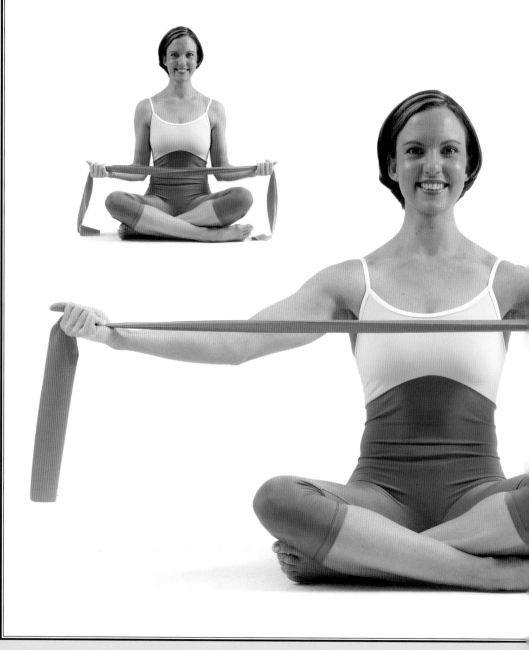

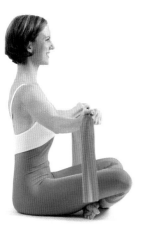

RHOMBOIDS

1 Sit tall, holding the stretchband looser now. Face the palms of your hands up.

2 As you exhale lengthen your arms as though you are presenting a long platter to someone. Keep your elbows slightly bent, your shoulders back, your abdominals lifted and your neck relaxed.

3 Inhale, relaxing your arms but keep your back and stomach strong.

4 Repeat 10–12 times.

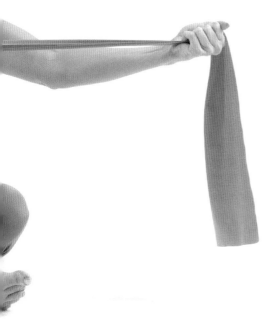

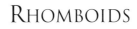

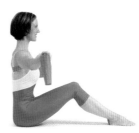

MODIFICATION

If you are finding it difficult to eliminate neck tension, try wrapping the stretchband around your upper back and under your armpits. Stretch your arms in a similar manner. Emphasise your abdominals lengthening and visualise yourself leaning flat against a wall.

SHOULDER & ARMWORK *(continued)*

OFFERING

1 Sit on the middle of the stretchband and hold the ends in your hands so that your thumbs point up during the exercise. Lengthen your spine and stabilise your shoulder blades.

2 As you exhale, pull your arms up at an angle slightly wider than your knees. Maintain a very strong torso, keeping the tension out of your neck as much as possible. Do not hitch your shoulders up in effort to raise your arms.

3 Inhale and relax, but don't slouch.

4 Repeat 6–10 times.

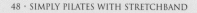

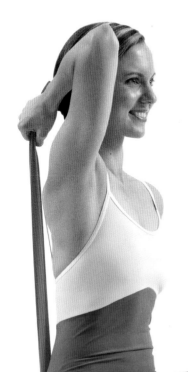

TRICEPS

1 Sit tall and hold the stretchband in one hand. Dangle it over your shoulder and catch it behind you with the other hand, anchoring it to your seat. Keep your high elbow pointing forward and your shoulders square to your front. Relax your neck and be careful not to arch your back.

2 As you exhale, raise your hand towards the ceiling maintaining the position of your upper arm. Ensure you don't hitch your shoulder up in effort to raise your hand.

3 Inhale and control your arm, bending again to challenge muscle control.

4 Repeat 10–12 times each arm.

Shoulder & Armwork *(continued)*

Triceps Extending

1 Sit with your legs together in front of you. Lean your body forward towards your thighs without slouching. Keep your stomach lifted and relax your neck, drawing your shoulders back. Sit on the stretchband, hold the ends and reach both arms out behind you, shoulder width apart.

2 As you exhale, lift your arms up behind you. Don't squeeze your shoulder blades together or go round shouldered. Keep scooping up your abdominals.

3 Inhale as you lower your arms again.

4 Repeat 10 times.

5 With calm breathing, pulse your arms up and down with short quick movements at the height of your shoulder range.

6 Repeat for 10–20 pulses.

7 Hold your arms as high as you can, without being round shouldered and bend and stretch your elbows for further tricep work.

8 Repeat 10 final extensions.

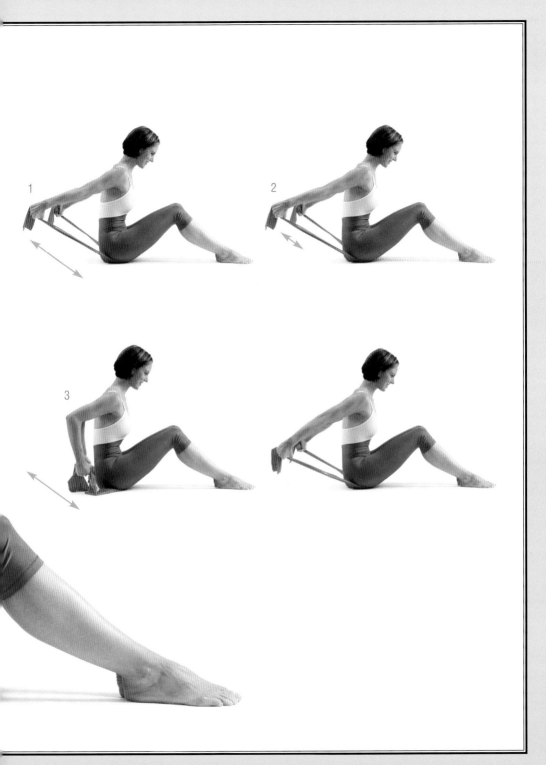

FULL-BODY INTEGRATION

Purpose: *To ultimately challenge your ability to have a whole-body focus while executing exercises that require stability of one part and movement of another. Often in Pilates you must feel opposing forces of resistance created by your own muscle effort in order to elongate, stabilise and move fluidly.*

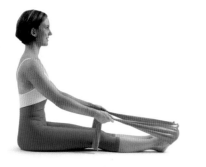

ROWING PREP (CHEST EXPANSION)

1 Sit upright with your legs straight in front of you (bent if you need to be able to sit taller without lower back strain). Place the stretchband around the balls of your feet and hold the ends with your hands. Lengthen your waist with strong, taut abdominals and lightly pull your shoulders back.

2 As you exhale, pull the stretchband and bend your arms next to your torso. Feel the breadth across your chest as your elbows reach back. Be careful not to lean backwards or use your neck.

3 Inhale as you release the band. Keep your abdominals lifted.

4 Repeat 10 times.

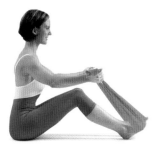

Rowing Prep
(Butterfly)

1 Sit as you were for Chest Expansion and hold the stretchband from beneath. You may have to lean forward a little and bend your knees.

2 As you exhale, pull your arms wide – only as far as you feel the muscles at the back of your shoulders, not your neck. Keep your stomach and upper back lengthened and strong.

3 Inhale as you release the band tension, but be careful not to slouch.

4 Repeat 5–10 times.

FULL BODY INTEGRATION *(continued)*

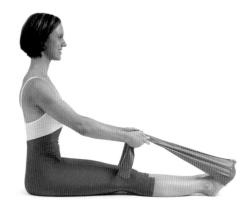

SPINAL ROTATION (ARCHERY)

1 Sit as you were for Rowing Prep with the stretchband around both feet.

2 Exhale as you pull one end of the stretchband and rotate your upper torso to that side. Keep your pelvis and legs still and use your oblique abdominals, together with the muscles of your upper back, to control the twist.

3 Inhale as you return to the front. Keep lengthening your abdominals and open your chest.

4 Repeat, alternating sides up to 10 times.

SPINAL ROTATION (SPINE TWIST)

1 Sit tall with both legs together and bent in front of you. Wrap the stretchband around your upper back and under your armpits. Hold on to the ends and stretch your arms to the sides. Maintain a lengthened spine and good shoulder position throughout.

2 As you exhale, rotate your upper torso with a double pulse action to one side.

3 Inhale, returning to the centre. Maintain a long waist.

4 Repeat, alternating sides for up to 10 times.

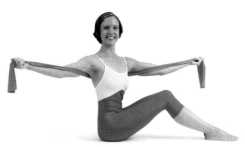

NOTE
Once you have stretched your arms to the sides, try to keep your shoulders and arms still with good posture throughout the exercise. The movement comes from your waist and middle-lower thoracic spine.

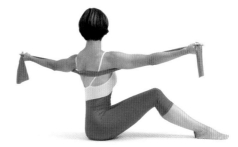

FULL BODY INTEGRATION *(continued)*

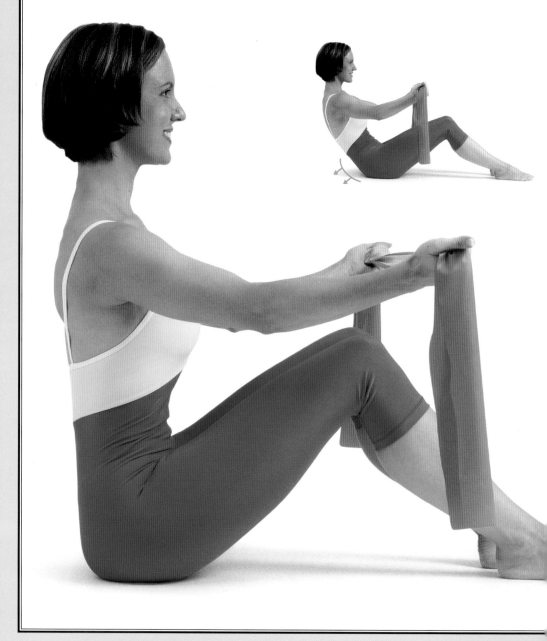

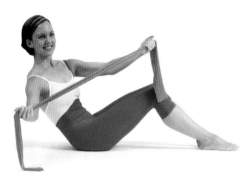

ROLL BACK WITH ROTATION

1 Sit as you did for Spine Twist, with your legs bent and slightly apart. Hold the stretchband in your hands, palms up, just wider than shoulder width. Keep some tension on the stretchband so that you are aware of your shoulder and upper back muscles. Scoop up through your abdominal muscles. Inhale.

2 As you exhale, pull your stomach to your spine and roll back to the point where you feel moderate challenge with your abdominals. Inhale. Hold still and continue to keep some tension on the stretchband.

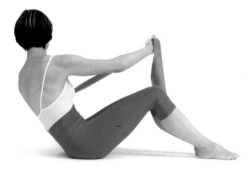

3 Exhale. Rotate your upper body without losing your deep abdominal work. Keep your pelvis and legs still. Inhale as you return to the centre, maintaining a stable pelvis and the same amount of roundness through the spine.

4 Exhale. Rotate to the other side. Inhale. Return to the centre.

5 Exhale. Roll forward towards your legs and sit tall.

6 Repeat 4–5 times.

STRETCHES

Purpose: *To release and elongate muscles that have been under tension or performing strength work. Combining strength, mobility and flexibility aspects to your exercise regime will promote a balanced physique.*

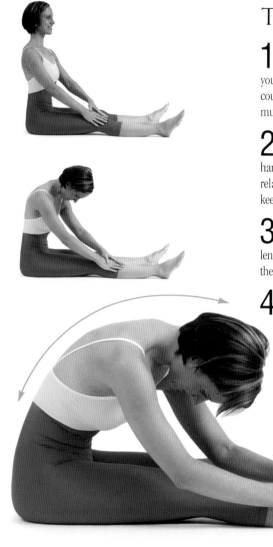

THORACIC RELEASE

1 Sit upright with your legs shoulder width apart, or slightly wider. If you are unable to sit tall with your legs straight, either bend your knees or sit on a couple of books. Lengthen your waist and abdominal muscles and breathe normally.

2 Place both hands on one leg and as you exhale, roll head-first towards your leg and slide your hands towards your shin. Ease into the stretch, relaxing both shoulders towards the floor. Try to keep the opposite hip anchored to the floor.

3 You may hold the stretch for 2–3 full breaths, then engage your deep abdominals as you roll up, lengthening your waist upright initially and rebuilding the spine piece-by-piece until you sit tall.

4 Repeat 4–6 times in total, alternating sides.

Psoas Stretch (Supine)

1 Lying on your back, place a cushion or rolled towel under the lowest part of your hips so that your lower back can still relax towards the floor. Hold one thigh up to the side of your chest, aiming for your shoulder. Lengthen your other leg along the floor.

2 Breathe normally and relax for 20–30 seconds.

3 Repeat on your other leg and repeat both again if the stretch feels beneficial for the front of your outstretched thigh and hip.

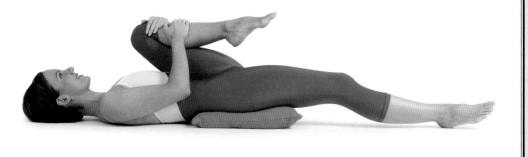

NOTE
The cushion or towel is optional, but will ensure a deeper hip flexor stretch.

STRETCHES *(continued)*

PSOAS STRETCH (KNEELING)

1 Kneel on one knee and lunge forward so that your weight is on your front heel and both hands. Ensure that both knees align with your shoulders so you don't go knock-kneed, and allow your back leg to relax so you feel the front of that hip stretching.

2 Hold for 20–30 seconds.

3 Repeat on your other leg and again on both legs.

NECK STRETCH

1 Sit upright. Keep your shoulders back and carefully tilt your head to one side – ear-to-shoulder – without allowing your shoulders to raise. You may need to stand in front of a mirror to see if you are keeping your shoulders level and that you are not rotating your neck and head.

2 Hold momentarily and repeat on the other side.

3 Repeat both sides.

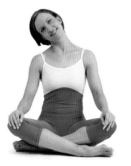

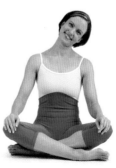

POWER PILATES
WORKOUT SEQUENCE (REFER DVD)

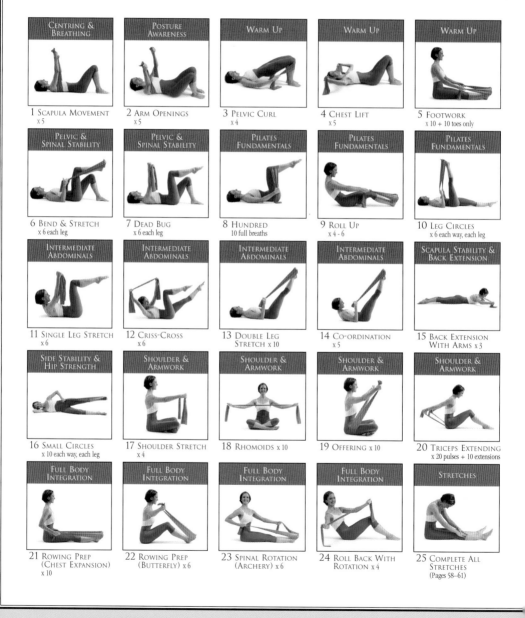

CENTRING & BREATHING
1 SCAPULA MOVEMENT
x 5

POSTURE AWARENESS
2 ARM OPENINGS
x 5

WARM UP
3 PELVIC CURL
x 4

WARM UP
4 CHEST LIFT
x 5

WARM UP
5 FOOTWORK
x 10 + 10 toes only

PELVIC & SPINAL STABILITY
6 BEND & STRETCH
x 6 each leg

PELVIC & SPINAL STABILITY
7 DEAD BUG
x 6 each leg

PILATES FUNDAMENTALS
8 HUNDRED
10 full breaths

PILATES FUNDAMENTALS
9 ROLL UP
x 4 - 6

PILATES FUNDAMENTALS
10 LEG CIRCLES
x 6 each way, each leg

INTERMEDIATE ABDOMINALS
11 SINGLE LEG STRETCH
x 6

INTERMEDIATE ABDOMINALS
12 CRISS-CROSS
x 6

INTERMEDIATE ABDOMINALS
13 DOUBLE LEG STRETCH x 10

INTERMEDIATE ABDOMINALS
14 CO-ORDINATION
x 5

SCAPULA STABILITY & BACK EXTENSION
15 BACK EXTENSION WITH ARMS x 3

SIDE STABILITY & HIP STRENGTH
16 SMALL CIRCLES
x 10 each way, each leg

SHOULDER & ARMWORK
17 SHOULDER STRETCH
x 4

SHOULDER & ARMWORK
18 RHOMOIDS x 10

SHOULDER & ARMWORK
19 OFFERING x 10

SHOULDER & ARMWORK
20 TRICEPS EXTENDING
x 20 pulses + 10 extensions

FULL BODY INTEGRATION
21 ROWING PREP (CHEST EXPANSION)
x 10

FULL BODY INTEGRATION
22 ROWING PREP (BUTTERFLY) x 6

FULL BODY INTEGRATION
23 SPINAL ROTATION (ARCHERY) x 6

FULL BODY INTEGRATION
24 ROLL BACK WITH ROTATION x 4

STRETCHES
25 COMPLETE ALL STRETCHES
(Pages 58–61)

GLOSSARY

ABDOMINAL MUSCLES
There are four layers of abdominal muscles. The six-pack crunches you forward; external and internal obliques (waist muscles) rotate and twist the torso with the internal obliques also assisting in trunk stabilisation; and the deeper layer (transversus abdominus) acts to stabilise the spine against any of these movements once the spine and pelvis is stable in a certain position. Transversus is often referred to as one of the core stabilisers.

GLUTEALS
The glutes are the muscle group of the buttocks, which contribute to hip movement and stabilisation of the pelvis and lower back.

HAMSTRINGS
The group of muscles at the back of the thigh which originate at the sitting bone and insert at the back of the knee. These help move the thigh backwards and/or bend the knee.

HIP FLEXORS
Muscles at the front of the hip (groin area), one of which is the psoas. They contract to lift the thigh to the torso. The psoas directly affect the lower back if tight and/or weak.

LATS (LATISSIMUS DORSI)
Large muscle of the back which engages as the arm draws backwards.

PECS (PECTORALIS MINOR/MAJOR)
Muscles of the chest and front of the shoulder which are commonly tight due to the amount of activity we do with the arms in front of our torsos, such as lifting objects.

PELVIC FLOOR
Thin layer of muscles suspended across the pelvic girdle which supports the weight of the abdominal organs and shares nerve connections with both deep abdominal muscles and the respiratory diaphragm. Activation of the pelvic floor contributes to strengthening of the abdominal region.

RHOMBOIDS
Muscles between the thoracic spine and the shoulder blades which contribute to scapula stabilisation for better posture.

ROTATOR CUFF
Four muscles comprise the rotator cuff which act synergistically to hold the shoulder joint stable and aligned.

SCAPULA (SCAPULAE — PLURAL)
The shoulder blade, which helps make up the shoulder joint, provides attachments for many of the upper back muscles. Stabilising the scapulae flat against the ribcage is essential for good posture.

SITTING BONES
These are the lowest boney protrusions of the pelvis that you are aware of when you sit on a hard surface. They provide an attachment site for the hamstrings, and when you sit exactly on them, or slightly behind them, you are usually in a neutral pelvic alignment.

SPINE
The spine is made up of different sections. The cervical spine is that of the neck; thoracic being the middle upper back and the attachment for all the ribs; the lumbar spine is that of the lower back; and the saccral and coccygeal are that of the pelvis and tailbone.

SUPINE
This is the anatomical term for lying on your back. Prone is when you are lying face down.

TRICEPS
These muscles are those of the back of the upper arm, running from the back of the shoulder to the elbow.

CONCLUSION

Joseph Pilates is considered to have been ahead of his time in his strategies for full-body strengthening and his analysis of overall healthy living. It is said that he continued to define, refine and challenge his philosophy of body conditioning throughout his years, endeavouring to assist individuals in overcoming physical limitations. Now, as modern physical science continues to discover more about how our muscles and joints move, Pilates Masters continue to evolve the movement which is based on Joseph's original teachings. However, the principles behind the movement will always remain the same and will continue to have great impact on the health and lives of those who practise Pilates.

Incorporating a stretchband into a Pilates workout creates a new dimension for you to enhance your experience with the Method. As you adopt routine Pilates practice into your life, you will discover a centredness and greater ease of movement. It is always important that you periodically return to the basics in order to understand how the fundamental principles completely affect the continuing benefits you will gain from this unique method of full-body conditioning.

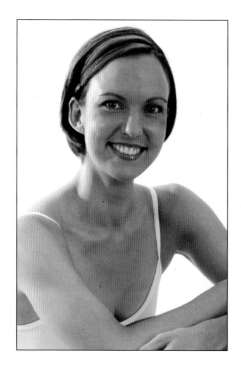

ABOUT THE AUTHOR

Jennifer Pohlman was first introduced to Pilates as a dance student while completing a Bachelor of Dance degree at the Victorian College of the Arts in Melbourne. She later trained as an instructor and taught the Pilates Method in Brisbane and Gold Coast studios before establishing her own Gold Coast studio at Kirra, called Pilates InsideOut. Jennifer's previous titles include *Simply Pilates, Simply Ball with Pilates Principles, The Complete Ball Workout with Pilates, The Complete Pilates on Mat* and *More Simply Pilates*.